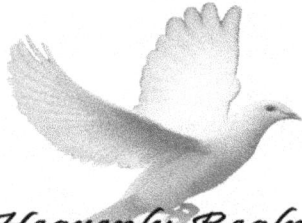

Heavenly Realm Publishing
Houston, Texas

Published By: Heavenly Realm Publishing
P. O. Box 682532, Houston, TX 77268
www.heavenlyrealmpublishing.com
Toll Free 1-866-216-0696

Printed in the United States of America

ISBN—13: 9781937911-90-4 (paperback)

Library of Congress Cataloging-in-Publication Data: 2015907757
Stephanie Franklin
REshape YOU Elderly Fitness Exercises & Eating Plan Book/ Stephanie Franklin

1. Health & Fitness: Exercise —United States. **2.** HEALTH & FITNESS/Diet &
Nutrition / General —United States. **3.** Health & Fitness: Healing —United States.

This book is printed on acid free paper.

Scripture quotations are from the Holy Bible. All rights reserved.

Stephanie Franklin
PO Box 682532
Houston, TX 77268
reshapeyou.stephaniefranklin.org

REshape YOU

Elderly Fitness

Fitness

Exercises & Eating Plan Book

A Fitness Book of Simple Exercises
& Eating Plans for the Elderly.

- ✓ Quick Weight Loss
- ✓ Simple Exercises in a Chair
- ✓ Simple Standing Exercises
- ✓ Simple Bed Exercises
- ✓ Simple Walking & Strength Training
- ✓ Motivational Tips
- ✓ Healthy Eating Plan
- ✓ Simple 5-Week Exercises & Eating Plan

The Whole-Body Benefits of
Exercises for Older Adults

Stephanie Franklin

*A Fitness Guide to Teach You How to Create
the **NEW YOU** from the Inside Out as an Older Adult.*

Achieve Greatness in **YOU** as an Older Adult!

REshape YOU

Elderly Fitness Exercises & Eating Plan Book

Contents:

FICTION NOVELS & MOTIVATIONAL BOOKS:

1. When Ramona Got Her Groove Back from God
2. My Song of Solomon
3. My Song of Solomon *Prayer Journal*
4. God Loves Thugs Too!
5. The Locker Room Experience: *For the Struggling Athlete & Coach, & Tips on How to Get Recruited in Sports*
6. REshape YOU: *A Fitness Guide to Teach You How to Create the NEW YOU from the Inside Out*
7. REshape YOU Elderly Fitness Exercises & Eating Plan Book

MINISTRY BOOKS & WORKBOOK:

8. Position Your Faith for Great Success
9. Position Your Faith for Great Success *Workbook*
10. The Purpose Chaser: *For Children Ages 5 to 12*
11. Church Hurt: *How to Heal & Overcome It*
12. The Power of Healing
13. The Power of the Holy Spirit
14. Winning Together: *His Needs Matter, Her Needs Are Important*
15. Winning Together as a Parent: *Loving Each Other While Knowing Your Children and Teen are Included and Not Separate.*

You may purchase them at any Christian Bookstore, Barnes & Noble, Amazon.com, Books-a-Million, Borders, and anywhere books are sold.

RE*shape* YOU

Fitness Elderly

Exercises & Eating Plan Book

A Fitness Book of Simple Exercises
& Eating Plans for the Elderly.

CONCERNS YOU MAY HAVE

- ➤ Are you concerned about your health?
- ➤ Want to learn how to have better eating habits?
- ➤ Concerned about falling?
- ➤ Concerned about having balance, mobility, and coordination?
- ➤ Want to stop procrastinating?
- ➤ Want the ability to participate in daily activities?
- ➤ Want to maintain or improve your functional level?
- ➤ Want to get in tiptop shape at your age?
- ➤ Want better eating habits?
- ➤ Want to learn how to do simple exercises at your age?
- ➤ Are you spiritually drained?
- ➤ Mental & emotional fatigue?
- ➤ Need and want a NEW look?

RE shape YOU Elderly Fitness & Exercises & Eating Plan Book will help answer questions and change all of your concerns. Read on…

PREFACE

REshape YOU for the Elderly

*This RE**shape** YOU book is designed* for the seasoned elderly who have many blessed years here on earth. As the years go by, you may think that you are getting old and chances are for you to stay and look healthy and in great bodily shape is none. You may have looked at different rigorous exercise books, videos, DVD's, and have almost attempted to try them yourself. However, as you may attempted to try them, your strength could not allow you to do them. This is why I have designed a <u>very simple exercise book</u> just for you that will help change you from the inside out. I have also included an eating plan (diet) that will help you as you successfully complete the simple exercises. Each exercise will help you:

1. Get your blood circulating
2. Help you lose weight the healthy way
3. Maintain bone density
4. Learn how to have great health
5. Reduce the risk of falling
6. Simple and light strength training exercises *(if you chose)*
7. Improve balance, mobility, and coordination
8. Regain the ability to participate in activities
9. Maintain or improve your functional level
10. Recover from bodily rehabilitation from injuries and surgery
11. Feel and look healthy while getting the activity of your limbs moving.

If you have someone who is able to move faster than you, they are encouraged to help assist you and/or even do the exercises with you. They will motivate and push you to complete the tasks. If you do not have anyone to assist you, you can still accomplish it alone.

I believe in you and I believe that you can do all things through God who gives you the strength and the help you need.

INTRODUCTION

REshape YOU for the Elderly

I wrote a fitness book called, "RE*shape* YOU: *A Fitness Guide to Teach You How to Create the* **NEW YOU** *from the Inside Out.*" As I was writing the book, and preparing the exercises and eating plans, I realized that the book may be too hard for those who are up in age. As I looked around to find books with exercises that cater to the seasoned elderly age, it was almost impossible to find. So, with that said, I have come up with this very easy, as I have stated before, step by step exercise book for the seasoned elderly who still wants to exercise, want to build strength, maintain healthy bone density, improve balance, mobility, and coordination, reduce the risk of falling, maintain independence of performing activities on a daily basis; and have healthy eating habits.

This book not only caters to exercises, but it does just what the book title states, it also deals with the elderly person who struggles with low self-esteem, depression, insecurities, and many other inner challenges that keep them from fulfilling the fitness and healthy eating goal they so desire.

RE*shape* YOU: *the Senior & Elderly Fitness Exercises & Eating Plan Book*, provides simple exercises and eating plans fit just for the elderly that target their age. It gives a breakdown of why exercising is important, it REshapes areas for improvement, such as:

1. Provides a stress reliever.
2. Brings peace of mind.
3. Takes pressure off the heart.
4. Provides a spiritual motivation and meditation in which the elderly is in need of.
5. It RE*shapes* YOU from the inside out, and creates a **NEW YOU**, that makes you feel like an entirely **NEW** person who can enjoy life to the fullest.

I am a firm believer that you cannot lose weight and live a healthy life without removing all of the inner stress build up from your past and from present issues (individual issues, or marital issues, or sibling issues, or family issues, or financial issues, the anxiety of aging issues, or job related issues, and/or more).

My goal is for everyone to experience the RE*shape* YOU experience from the inside out by participating in what this book has to offer.

Making the Change for Yourself

✓ Aging Changes
✓ Making the Change for Yourself
✓ Motivate Yourself
✓ The Power is Within You

Change is always hard especially when it has to do with age. It can be very challenging and at most times, most people never want to deal with it until it becomes necessary.

Making a positive change for yourself can be a challenge whether young or older. Unfortunately, none of us have a choice as to whether or not we want to get older. We all increase in number each year of our lives. The most powerful thing that each of us can do is enjoy every one of them to the fullest as they come.

As older adults increase in age, many challenges can set in like: aging changes in bones, muscles, joints, skin, hair, heart, mind, body, and soul if not monitored and if a health plan is not in place. For example, on the eating side: I am speaking of changing the way you cook your foods like not frying your foods, but baking them instead. Also staying away from sugar added foods, junk foods, sodas and punch. On the exercise side: I am speaking of you getting involved in a consistent exercise plan. As I just stated, many challenges can set in if not taken into consideration. Look below as I give some detailed examples:

✓ **AGING CHANGES**

- Bone density is lost as you age, especially in women after menopause. The bone loses calcium along with other ailments. The vertebrae (the spine) becomes weaker and begins to slump over.

- The muscles turn into fat, which brings flab under arms, neck, stomach, and thighs. Also causes lost in muscle tissue. Aging changes in the muscles become rigid with age and may lose tone. With regular exercise, this can be deleted and can even be minimized.

- The joints get stiffer and less flexible. Hip and knee joints may begin to lose joint cartilage. The finger joints lose cartilage and the bones thicken slightly.

- The skin begins to sag.

- The hair turns grey.

- The **HEART** can become weaker if a healthy daily exercise and healthy eating plan (diet) is not in place. Also, the heart deals with more than just on the health side, it also deals with inner breakdowns such as: contrariness- disobedience, stubbornness, rebelliousness, uncooperativeness, alzheimer's, and more. The change in hormones also occur. Hormones can affect the attitude and bring a change in reaction, personality, and also in lifestyle. I have also found that when there are issues within the heart that have not been dealt with, will make the older adult live their life dealing with past hurts, guilt's, resentments, loneliness, the feeling that no one loves you, unhappy about how you are treated, feeling unappreciated, and do not believe that he or she can live life to the fullest as a healthy older adult. It also makes you not want to be bothered with anyone, not even with family. You have this feeling of just wanting to be alone no matter if it is the holiday or not. These issues can hinder your success in your daily exercise, healthy eating, and in your Spiritual walk. You will literally shut down, if you get started at all, and you will gain the weight back you've worked so hard to lose. It is so important to release these past and/or present issues through prayer and discussing them with others (spouse, child/children, family, friends, counselor, pastor, etc.) in order to have a peaceful and successful RE*shape* YOU healthy life.

- The **MIND** plays a big part in how an older adult thinks. As I have mentioned in my RE*shape* YOU: *A Fitness Guide to Teach You How to Create the NEW YOU from the Inside Out* book as well. It is important to have a mental health plan in place when the mind wants to shut down and not want to do anything. You have to literally speak to your mind and not allow it to control you or your actions and decisions. You have to literally tell it, "I am strong and **not** weak", "I will live and **not** die", "I will get my life back that has been lost", "I will **not** look at my age, I will lose weight and get myself in great shape", "I will get active and enjoy my life and **not** give up", "I will **not** starve myself and give up, I will eat healthy and live healthy", "I will control my eating and make it a way of life".

- The **BODY** is the most important asset of our being. The body is our temple. When the body shuts down, you completely shut down. When the body is healthy and strong, it brings positive attitudes and moods. It makes you feel free and full of energy and life. It will make you feel like you can do anything.

- In representing the **SOUL**, I am speaking in reference to the older adult who needs spiritual guidance. Spiritual guidance is important to regain all of the areas you are desiring as you age in having a healthy life and keeping it. When the soul is catered to, you will go through every day in spiritual meditation and devotion with God. You will keep this same spiritual mindset throughout your day as you get involve in daily activities. I have stated this in my REshape YOU: *A Fitness Guide to Teach You How to Create the NEW YOU from the Inside Out* book as well. Pray and believe that you can lose weight and have a healthy life and keep it.

✓ MAKING THE CHANGE FOR YOURSELF

The fact that you are reading this book, proves that you have decided to take the step to RE*shape* YOUR life. You have chosen to make a positive change in living a healthy life. You have decided to opt in and change how you act, think, and believe in yourself. You have chosen to take the limits off and are determined to look, feel, and act better.

Making the change for yourself means that you no longer live in the past and hold all of the hidden scars, past guilt's, resentments of what you did and did not do, sicknesses, past hurts, etc. You are completely determined to experience the RE*shape* YOU experience—a change from the inside out.

As you grab a hold of the RE*shape* YOU NEW life—the healthy wholesome life, you will not only notice and see positive physical changes as your clothes fit much better, you are not tired just walking around your home, you're stronger, energetic, and motivated to exercise daily and make your healthy eating plan a way of life.

✓ MOTIVATE YOURSELF

As you age, the thought of it can be the only thing on your mind. I have experienced this with elderly family and friends who have said the same. If this is you to, my encouragement to you is to learn to motivate yourself. You cannot wait for others to motivate you and make you feel young again. It takes you remembering the accomplishments you have made throughout the years and feast on them. Do not think about the negative letdowns from the past or even now, only think about the awesome achievements you've made, and let that be your motivation. You may have been a great athlete, or an avid reader who read books on a regular basis, or a loving person who has helped many people along the way. Whatever your accomplishments were, feast on them and do not worry about where your future is going, let it take care of itself. Let tomorrow be tomorrow. I have found that when you do this, it brings a world of peace and there is no room for depression, unhappiness, loneliness, fear, and the feeling of defeat that you cannot be a better person or have a NEW RE*shape* YOU life of determination to live a healthy life style.

✓ THE POWER IS WITHIN YOU

There are a million reasons one can find to not believe in the power that lies within yourself. It is very easy to judge negatively rather than positively. The world is full of it. People generally feed off of each other whether negative or positive but more negative than anything. Has this ever been you? This type of energy transfers on you if you allow it to. It works especially when all you see or hear is negative. The transformation is easy. This is the goal to captivate your mind to think of yourself negatively and your life negatively, and also not believe that there is no possible way you can still get in tiptop shape at your age.

The power that is within you is not some superficial power. It is real, and it is the power that God has given to you to achieve, to excel, to prosper, to be strong, and all that you want to be. You will find that you can do anything with this power. Everything just comes together. Do you agree? Have you found this person to be you now or at one point in time in your life? Explain below.

_____

_____

_____

_____

_____

_____

_____

I challenge you to reach for the power that is within you and let that power be your guide and motivation to create the NEW YOU—the RE*shape* YOU person. Try it. It works. Feed off of the positive energy and not the negative energy. The power is already within you.

Making the Change as a Family

✓ Making the Change as a Family

As a loved one ages, and the effects of aging occur, it can be a challenge for the family to cope with.

Here are some steps on how to cope with the change in aging of a parent, loved one, or friend:

1. Take each day at a time.
2. Do not play into their negative words and feed backs, if any. But replace them with words of love and positive motivation.

3. Watch what you say and how you speak to them. Do not make their aging a negative thing rather than a beautiful seasoned thing.

4. Remove past issues that you are not happy with concerning them.

5. Be ready to forgive them for any mistakes they may make due to memory lapse and/or mood swings due to aging.

6. Always offer to help wherever needed and make them feel loved and not old.

7. Be patient with them and do not rush them.

8. Do not disrespect or treat them rough.

9. Enjoy the precious time you have with them. Make everyday a fun life filled moment for you (all).

10. Get out and exercise or enjoy a fun activity together.

11. Eat healthy together.

12. Go on fun trips together.

13. Enjoy life. Enjoy each other.

14. Love life. Love each other.

Here are some steps on how to cope with the change in yourself as an elderly and older adult, and as you are around family, children, and friends:

1. Do not make their visiting you a miserable one. Enjoy every minute you share with them.
2. Remove any complaining.
3. Embrace them with so much love and appreciation.
4. Remove the woe-its-me syndrome. And the "I am so old" attitude. You are not old unless you receive that you are old. It is important to keep a motivating and positive attitude at all times and watch your words. This will make you feel stronger.
5. Understand that getting a proper exercise and eating healthy is not an option, it is a way of life.
6. Live each day enjoying your life with them exercising or enjoying a fun activity day.

If you have an elderly parent, loved one, or friend, it is important to encourage them to eat healthy and exercise. You can even exercise with them and join in with them to eat healthy meals per day. It will not only be healthy for them, but it will be healthy for the both of you. You can also encourage them to get on board, get up, and get going to begin their exercising and new eating plan life style as I have provided in this RE*shape* YOU book. They are simple and an effective fit just for the one in need. Read along and lets begin...

ITEMS NEEDED FOR THE DAILY EXERCISES

Before you begin the simple daily exercises and eating plan in this book, you will need number's 1-12. If you do not have these items, don't worry, you can still do them anyway.

1. Faith, mental, motivation, and determination to do whatever it takes to RE*shape* yourself from the inside out.
2. Chair, exercise mat, bed, or couch.
3. 1, 2, or 3 pound hand weights (dumbbells) *(If weights/dumbbells are too heavy, you can complete the exercises without them. If weights/dumbbells are too light, you can increase the weight).*
4. Workout gloves *(if you so desire).*
5. 8 oz bottle or cup of water.
6. T-Shirt or comfortable shirt.
7. Walking shorts, or comfortable shorts or comfortable warm-ups.
8. Socks.
9. Exercise shoes *(tennis shoes or walking shoes).*
10. Gym bag *(if needed).*
11. Towel.

PLEASE BE ADVISED

Although the simple exercises in this book are very simple and harmless, please be advised that each exercise still may be too rigorous for some. Each level of exercises in this book are not intended to hurt, harm, or injure those who try them. If you feel that they are too rigorous, please consult your physician or those who assist you before beginning.

CHOOSE YOUR LEVEL

Before beginning, please pick the level you are on below, and follow that level throughout the book.

EXERCISE LEVEL ADD ✓ BELOW	
1. Beginners Level	
2. Immediate Level	
3. Senior Pro Level	

As you begin the simple exercises & eating plan, you may write your daily exercises & eating progress and goals below.

MY DAILY EXERCISES & EATING PLAN CHART:
• MONDAY
• TUESDAY
• WEDNESDAY
• THURSDAY
• FRIDAY
• SATURDAY
• SUNDAY

Now that you have chosen your level, and are ready to write down your eating plan information, you are now ready to begin.

Ready? LET'S GET STARTED...

CHAPTER 1 Walking
Exercises

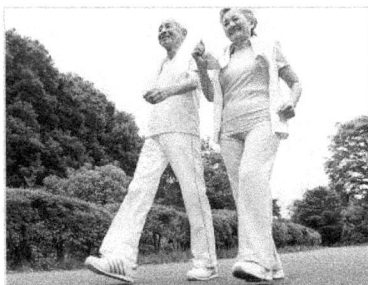

Beginners Walking

Before beginning, if you are unable to walk a long distance or at all, you may either walk in place or do the walking exercises in bed by pulling your knees upward and downward as if you are walking. I will explain this process more in detail below. Are you ready? Let's get started...

The Beginners Walking is for the Senior Elderly who is unable to walk but can move your legs. You may be confined to a bed and cannot get out of the bed. I have provided an exercise just for you below. It is very simple and as you continue to do them, you may even move up to the Immediate Level very soon. The goal is to get stronger and move up to the highest level. I encourage you to do your best and please do it with a positive attitude as you increase your faith and determination. You may have an assistant or you may do these by yourself. Take your time, you do not have to rush, rushing will only injure you. But, when you take your time and do them right, it will be rewarding for you. Just do not quit. You can do it... Let's go!

Items Needed:
Nothing

REMEMBER	You may either lay down, sit down, stand up and walk in place using a chair for stability, or you may walk out doors. Take it slow until you get your strength to move faster. Follow the instructions for the Beginning, Immediate, and Senior Pro Walking Exercises.

If by some chance you are unable to do all of the exercises within the level you chose, it is okay, just do the ones that you can and do the best you can. You may get an assistant to help you if needed.

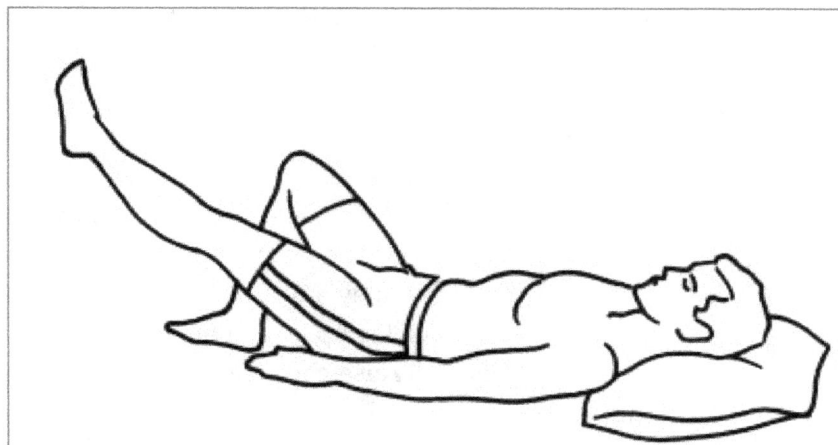

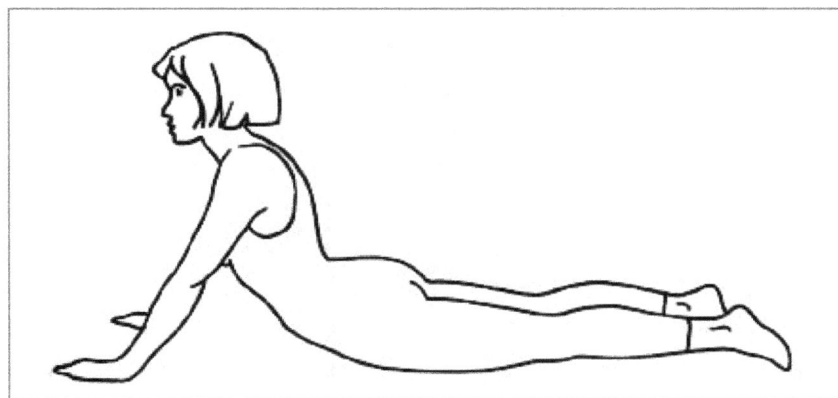

START EXERCISES

✓ BEGINNERS WALKING

1. **EXERCISE 1:** Tighten lower abs (stomach) to flatten back, slowly raise straight leg 8-12 inches or as high as you can off the floor or bed. If raising leg(s) is too hard, you may have someone assist you by them raising your leg up as you also try to do it with them. They will raise each leg up and down 3-5 times. For 3-sets total.

2. **EXERCISE 2:** Lay on your stomach. Press up on your hands slowly, keeping hips in contact with floor or bed. Relax low back and buttocks. You will do this for 3-5 times for 3-sets total.

3. **EXERCISE 3:** As you lay in the bed, stretch both legs straight out as you bring them together. You will then pull your right leg upward toward your chest as far as you can and then push it back down while bringing your left leg upward to do the same thing as the right leg. If this is too hard, you may do them one at a time and bring them up as far as you can. You may have someone to assist you in doing this exercise. You will do this exercise 3-5 times with each leg for a total of 3 sets with 1 minute rest.

Repeat for 3-5 days per week. You may extend the days if desired.

4. **EXERCISE 4:** You will need an assistant for this exercise. Your assistant will slightly grab the back of your ankle with their left hand, while holding your toes with their right hand and slowly turn the top of the foot in a clockwise direction for a total of 2-3 full turns, and repeat it by turning them in the opposite direction. The assistant will repeat this with each ankle for 3 sets of 2-3 turns with 30 sec rest in between. You may increase the turns as you desire, but do not exceed beyond what you can handle. Gloves may be used in this process.

Immediate Walking

The Immediate Walking is for the Senior and Elderly who is able to walk but your strength will not allow you to walk very far or for a long distance. I have provided a couple of exercises just for you under the "START EXERCISES" below. They are very simple exercises, and as you continue to do them, you may even move up to the Senior Pro Level very soon. The goal is to move up to the highest level. I encourage you to do your best and please do it with a positive attitude as you increase your faith and determination. You may have an assistant or you may do these by yourself. Take your time, you do not have to rush, rushing will only injure you. But, when you take your time and do them right, it will be rewarding for you. Just do not quit. You can do it... Let's go!

> **Items Needed:**
> 1. Stop watch or watch with a second hand, or you may count out loud
> 2. Sweat towel
> 3. Walking shoes
> 4. Socks
> 5. Shorts or warm ups
> 6. T-Shirt or comfortable shirt
> 7. You may listen to music as you do this

START EXERCISES

✓ IMMEDIATE WALKING

1. **EXERCISE 1:** You will position yourself at one end of the room and will walk to the other end of the room as fast as you can. The room or space needs to be at least 8-10 feet in length with enough room to turn around. You will then repeat this on a timed schedule. You will walk back and forth for 2 minutes. After 2 minutes, you will then stop and rest for 2-5 minutes and then proceed with the next set. You will have a total of 5 sets. If your room is much too small, you may do this exercise in your front yard, back yard, at your local park, or where ever you will have enough room. As you walk, you will move your arms in a runner's motion as if to be running but you are walking. It is also called a power walk. Your walking and arm movement is in unison. You will repeat this for 3 to 5 days. You may extend the days if desire. If you desire to extend your days, you will need to increase the minutes on each exercise each week you continue.

2. **EXERCISE 2:** You will do walking lunges. You will step as far as you can while bending your knees as much as possible in unison. You do not have to

go all the way down to the ground unless you can. All will need to do is step and lunge as you do this to the other side of the room, space, or area you provided. You will do this for a total of 2 minutes. After 2 minutes, you will then rest for 30 seconds to 1 minute and then proceed with the next set. You will have a total of 3-5 sets depending on the maximum strength you have. 3 sets is the minimum. Your arms should be extending forward a long with the opposite leg. You will repeat this for seven days. You may extend the days if desire.

Senior Pro Walking

The Senior Pro Walking is for the Senior and Elderly who is able to power walk for a long distance. Power walking is walking at a fast rate of speed. It is almost like running but you are still in a fast walking mode. I have provided a couple of exercises just for you below. They are very simple and as you continue to do them, you may even want to increase your walking distance and minutes very soon. The goal is to go higher and higher. I encourage you to do your best and please do it with a positive attitude as you increase your faith and determination. You may have an assistant or you may do these by yourself. Take your time, you do not have to rush, rushing will only injure you. But, when you take your time and do them right, it will be rewarding for you. Just do not quit. You can do it... Let's go!

Items Needed:
1. Stop watch or watch with a second hand
2. Sweat towel
3. Walking shoes
4. Socks
5. Shorts or warm ups

6. T-Shirt or comfortable shirt
7. You may listen to music as you do this

START EXERCISES

✓ SENIOR PRO WALKING

1. **EXERCISE:** You will either walk down to the end of your street and back, around the block in your neighborhood and back, around a/the track, or at a local park. You will power walk for a total of 10-15 minutes and then rest for 5-10 minutes. After you have rested for 5-10 minutes, you will proceed to the last set. You will then start the power walk again for another 10-15 minutes. After you have completed the second power walk, you will have completed the exercise. You will have a total of 2 sets *(power walks)*. As you walk, you will move your arms in a runner's motion as if to be running but you are walking at a fast pace. Your walking and arm movement is in unison. You will repeat this for 4-5 days. You may extend the days if desire. If you desire to extend your days, you will need to increase the minutes on each exercise each week you continue. Remember your rest time.

2. **EXERCISE 2:** You will power walk for 20-30 minutes by either walk down to the end of your street and back, around the block in your neighborhood and back, around a/the track, or at

a local park. You will power walk for a total of 20-30 minutes and then rest for 10-15 minutes. After you have rested for 10-15 minutes, you will proceed to the last set. You will then start the power walk again for another 20-30 minutes. After you have completed the second power walk, you will have completed the exercise. You will have a total of 2 sets *(power walks)*. As you walk, you will move your arms in a runner's motion as if to be running but you are walking at a fast pace. Your walking and arm movement is in unison. You will repeat this for 4-5 days. You may extend the days if desire. If you desire to extend your days, you will need to increase the minutes on each exercise each week you continue. Remember your rest time.

Now that you have completed the Walking Exercises and got your starting experience, you should challenge yourself to go a little further by starting and finishing the 5-Week Exercise & Eating Plan located in Chapter 6. I encourage you to start and finish it successfully.

CHAPTER 2 Sitting
Exercises

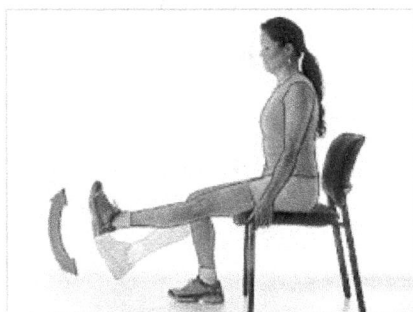

Beginners Sitting

Before beginning, please make sure you have all of the items and equipment that is needed. This will require a chair for sitting. Are you ready? Let's get started...

The Beginners Sitting is for the Senior/Elderly who is unable to walk far, or just would like to do sitting exercises. Below, I have provided several exercises just for you. They are very simple and as you continue to do them, you may even move up to the Immediate Level very soon. The goal is to move up to the highest level. I encourage you to do your best and please do it with a positive attitude as you increase your faith and determination. You may have an assistant or you may do these by yourself. Take your time, you do not have to rush, rushing will only injure you. But, when you take your time and do them right, it will be rewarding for you. Just do not quit. You can do it... Let's go!

Items Needed:

1. Sweat towel
2. Walking shoes
3. Socks
4. Shorts or warm ups
5. T-Shirt or comfortable shirt
6. A sitting chair
7. You may listen to music as you do this

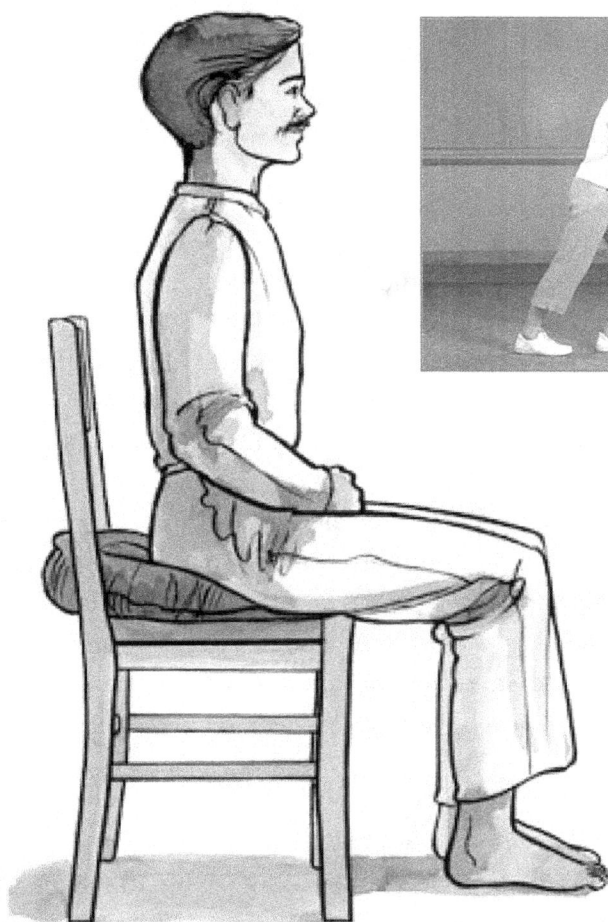

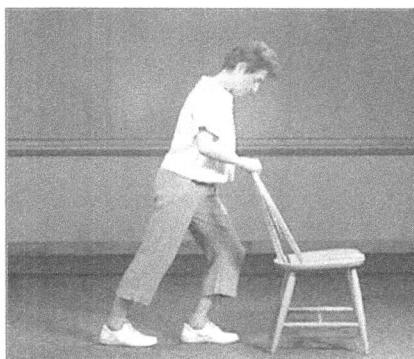

REMEMBER Relax as you breathe through each repetition and each exercise. Keep your back straight and do not slump down. Follow the instructions for the Sitting Exercises on the next page.

START EXERCISES

✓ BEGINNERS SITTING

1. **EXERCISE 1:** You will sit in a chair. You will then sit straight up and slightly lift your knee up and forward and tap the ground with your right toe as you repeat the process with the left toe. You will tap your right and left toe as you slightly lift up your knee for a total of 4-6 times. After you complete the taps, you will then rest for 30-seconds to 1 minute. After you have rested, you will then repeat this process again for 2-3 sets, as you do them 4-6 more times. You will repeat this process for 2-4 days. You may extend the days if desire. If you desire to extend your days, you will need to increase the amount of times on each exercise each week you continue.

2. **EXERCISE 2:** You will sit in a chair. You will then extend both feet outward as straight as possible. You will then hold each side of the chair with your right and left hands tightly as you grip each side. You will then pull your legs upward toward your chest. You will come up as high as possible and then stretch them back out until your legs are straight again for a count of 5 times. You will repeat this process for 3-5 sets. If using two legs

at one time are too hard, you may use one leg at a time as you repeat the process the same amount of times. If your legs are strong and lifting two legs at one time is still too light, you may want to add ankle weights on each ankle for extra weight. You will repeat this process for 3-5 days. You may extend the days if desire. If you desire to extend your days, you will need to increase the amount of times on each exercise each week you continue.

Immediate Sitting

The Immediate Sitting is for the Senior/Elderly who is unable to walk far, or just would like to do sitting exercises. I have provided a couple of exercises just for you below. They are very simple and as you continue to do them, you may even move up to the Senior Pro Level very soon. The goal is to get stronger and move up to the highest level. I encourage you to do your best and please do it with a positive attitude as you increase your faith and determination. You may have an assistant or you may do these by yourself. Take your time, you do not have to rush, rushing will only injure you. But, when you take your time and do them right, it will be rewarding for you. Just do not quit. You can do it... Let's go!

Items Needed:
1. Sweat towel
2. Walking shoes
3. Socks
4. Shorts or warm ups
5. T-Shirt or comfortable shirt
6. Large matt or large towel
7. A sitting chair
8. You may listen to music as you do this

START EXERCISES

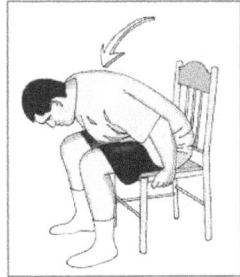

✓ IMMEDIATE SITTING

1. **EXERCISE 1:** You will sit in a chair and will tightly grip both sides of the chair with your hands. Look at the diagram above. You will then bend downward almost placing your face on your thighs. If you cannot bend that far down, go as far as you can. You will repeat this process 4-6 times and rest for 2 minutes. You will repeat the process again for a total of 3-5 sets. You will repeat this process for 5 days. You may extend the days if desire. If you desire to extend your days, you will need to increase the amount of times on each exercise each week you continue.

2. **EXERCISE 2:** You will sit in a chair and will tightly grip both sides of the chair with your hands. You will then extend your legs outward,

keeping them bent in an "L" shape appearance—right leg at a bent position going toward the right, left leg going toward the left. You will then close and then open your legs as quickly as possible, keeping them at a bent position. You will repeat this process 3-5 times and will rest for 2 minutes. You will repeat the process again for a total of 3 sets. You will repeat this process for 3-5 days. You may extend the days if desire. If you desire to extend your days, you will need to increase the amount of times on each exercise each week you continue.

Senior Pro Sitting

The Senior Pro Sitting is for the Senior/Elderly who is able to walk far and would like to do sitting exercises. I have provided a couple of exercises just for you below. They are very simple and as you continue to do them, you may even want to increase your walking distance and minutes very soon. The goal is to go higher and higher. I encourage you to do your best and please do it with a positive attitude as you increase your faith and determination. You may have an assistant or you may do these by yourself. Take your time, you do not have to rush, rushing will only injure you. But, when you take your time and do them right, it will be rewarding for you. Just do not quit. You can do it... Let's go!

Items Needed:
1. Sweat towel
2. Walking shoes or comfortable shoes
3. Socks
4. Shorts or warm ups
5. T-Shirt or comfortable shirt
6. A sitting chair
7. You may listen to music as you do this

START EXERCISES

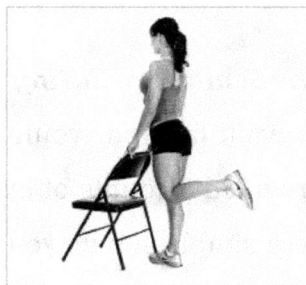

✓ SENIOR PRO SITTING

1. <u>**EXERCISE 1:**</u> You will stand behind your chair and place your hands on the back of the chair. You will then tiptoe with both feet at the same time, tiptoe as high as you can and drop down as you repeat the process 5-10 times. You will then rest for 30 seconds to 1 minute and then repeat the process for 3-5 sets. You may increase the amount of times and the sets as you get stronger or as needed. You will also repeat this process for 3-5 days. You may extend the days if desire. If you desire to extend your days, you will need to increase the amount of times and sets on each exercise each week you continue.

2. <u>**EXERCISE 2:**</u> You will stand behind your chair and place your hands on the back of the chair.

You will then lift your right foot backwards in an upward position. You will lift your right leg 5-10 times and repeat the same process with your left leg the same amount of times. You will repeat both leg exercises for 3-5 sets. You may increase the amount of times and the sets as you get stronger or as needed. You will also repeat this process for 5 days. You may extend the days if desire. If you desire to extend your days, you will need to increase the amount of times and sets on each exercise each week you continue.

Now that you have completed the Sitting Exercises and got your starting experience, you should challenge yourself to go a little further by starting and finishing The 5-Week Exercise & Eating Plan located in Chapter 6. I encourage you to start and finish it successfully.

CHAPTER 3   Arms
Exercises

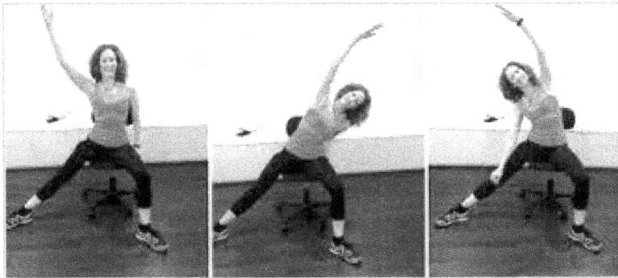

Beginners Arms

Before beginning, please make sure you have all of the items and equipment that is needed. This will require a chair for sitting. Are you ready? Let's get started...

The Beginners Arms is for the Senior/Elderly who is able to do arm exercises. Below, I have provided a couple of exercises just for you. They are very simple and as you continue to do them, you may even move up to the Immediate Level very soon. The goal is to move up to the highest level. I encourage you to do your best and please do it with a positive attitude as you increase your faith and determination. You may have an assistant or you may do these by yourself. Take your time, you do not have to rush, rushing will only injure you. But, when you take your time and do them right, it will be rewarding for you. Just do not quit. You can do it... Let's go!

Items Needed:

1. Sweat towel
2. Walking shoes
3. Socks
4. Shorts or warm ups
5. T-Shirt or comfortable shirt
6. You may listen to music as you do this

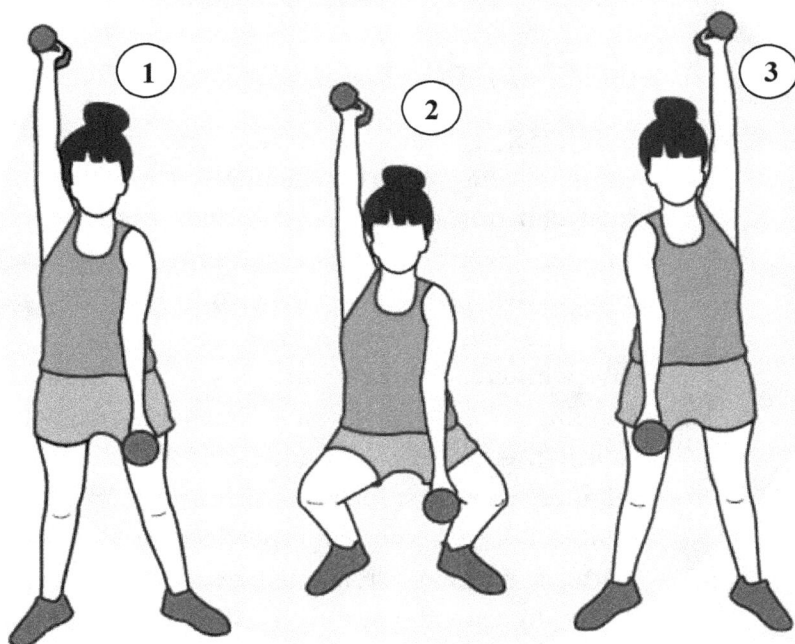

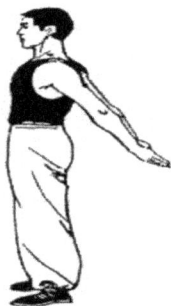

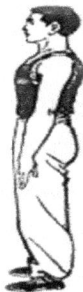

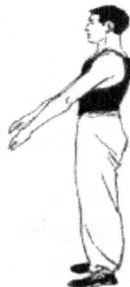

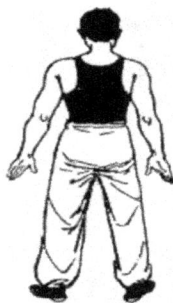

REMEMBER	Stand tall with both feet planted, and do not slouch or lock your knees. Follow the instructions for the Arm Exercises on the next page.

START EXERCISES

✓ BEGINNERS ARMS

1. **EXERCISE 1:** You will stand with your legs straddled and your arms extended outward to the right and to the left. You will then lower them straight down to your side and bring your right and left arms straight up over your heads into a clap. You will then lower them as quick as you can without moving your legs. Kind of like jumping jacks but not using your legs. You will repeat this process 3-5 times and rest for 1-2 minutes. You will repeat the process again for a total of 3-5 sets. You will repeat this process for 3-5 days. You may extend the days if desire. If you desire to extend your days, you will need to increase the amount of times on each exercise each week you continue.

2. **EXERCISE 2:** You will stand up or sit in a chair. You will punch forward with your right and left fist. You <u>may</u> use a 1, 2, 3, or 5 pound hand dumbbell/weight, depending on your strength. You will repeat this process 3-5 times and rest for 1-2 minutes. You will repeat the process again for a total of 3 sets. You will repeat this process for 3-5 days. You may extend the days if desire. If you

desire to extend your days, you will need to increase the amount of times on each exercise each week you continue.

Immediate Arms

The Immediate Arms is for the Senior/Elderly who is able to walk but your strength will not allow you to for a medium to long distance. I have provided a couple of exercises just for you below. They are very simple and as you continue to do them, you may even move up to the Senior Pro Level very soon. The goal is to move up to the highest level. I encourage you to do your best and please do it with a positive attitude as you increase your faith and determination. You may have an assistant or you may do these by yourself. Take your time, you do not have to rush, rushing will only injure you. But, when you take your time and do them right, it will be rewarding for you. Just do not quit. You can do it... Let's go!

Items Needed:
1. Sweat towel
2. Walking shoes
3. Socks
4. Shorts or warm ups
5. T-Shirt or comfortable shirt
6. Large matt or large towel
7. You may listen to music as you do this

START EXERCISES

✓ IMMEDIATE ARMS

1. **EXERCISE 1:** You will stand and straddle your legs as wide as you can. You will then lunge and reach to the right as far as you can and then lunge and reach to the left as far as you can 5-8 times. You will rest for 1-3 minutes. You will repeat the process again for a total of 3-5 sets. You will repeat this process for 3-5 days. You may extend the days if desire. If you desire to extend your days, you will need to increase the amount of times on each exercise each week you continue.

2. **EXERCISE 2:** You will stand or sit in a chair and as your feet are set in a stands or sitting position, you will use two 1, 2, 3, 5, or 8 pound dumbbells/hand weights, as you take your pick according to your strength. You will then curl each dumbbell/hand weight in each hand at the same time as you curl/bring them toward your chest and back down to your side for a 5-10 count. You will repeat this process for 3-5 sets. You will repeat this process for 3-5 days. You may also do this exercise without dumbbells/hand weights. All you will do is ball your left and right fist and curl them upward to your chest and back

down to your waist, to repeat the same process as you would if you had dumbbells in your hand. You may extend the days if desire. If you desire to extend your days, you will need to increase the amount of times on each exercise each week you continue.

Senior Pro Arms

The Senior Pro Arms is for the Senior/Elderly who is able to power walk for a long distance. Power walking is walking at a fast rate of speed. It is almost like running but you are still in a fast pace walking mode. I have provided a couple of exercises just for you below. They are very simple and as you continue to do them, you may even want to increase your walking distance and minutes very soon. The goal is to go higher and higher. I encourage you to do your best and please do it with a positive attitude as you increase your faith and determination. You may have an assistant or you may do these by yourself. Take your time, you do not have to rush, rushing will only injure you. But, when you take your time and do them right, it will be rewarding for you. Just do not quit. You can do it... Let's go!

Items Needed:
1. Sweat towel
2. Walking shoes
3. Socks
4. Shorts or warm ups
5. T-Shirt or comfortable shirt

6. Chair
7. Large matt or large towel
8. You may listen to music as you do this

START EXERCISES

✓ SENIOR PRO ARMS

1. **EXERCISE 1:** You will sit in a chair, on a matt, or on a large towel. You will then raise your arms in a running motion and move them as fast as you can as if to be running, for 5-15 seconds, non-stop. 5 is the minimum, you can increase your time if you like but you cannot go lower than the 5 seconds. You will then rest for 30-50 seconds. You will then repeat the process for 3-5 sets. You may increase the time and the sets as you get stronger or as needed. You will also repeat this process for 3-5 days. You may extend the days if desire. If you desire to extend your days, you will need to increase the amount of times and sets on each exercise each week you continue.

2. **EXERCISE 2:** You will sit in a chair or stand. You will then take two 1, 2, 3, 5, or 8 pound dumbbells/hand weights, as you take your pick according to your strength in each hand. As you have each dumbbell/hand weight in each hand, you will punch downward toward your side, punch outward from your chest, and then punch upward as you punch with each hand. You will repeat this process for 3-5 times. 3 is the

minimum, you can increase your time if you like but you cannot go lower than the 3. You will then rest for 1 minute. You will then repeat the process for 3-5 sets. You may increase the time and the sets as you get stronger or as needed. You will also repeat this process for 3-5 days. You may extend the days if desire. If you desire to extend your days, you will need to increase the amount of times and sets on each exercise each week you continue.

Now that you have completed the Arms Exercises and got your starting experience, you should challenge yourself to go a little further by starting and finishing The 5-Week Exercise & Eating Plan located in Chapter 6. I encourage you to start and finish it successfully.

CHAPTER 4 Legs
Exercises

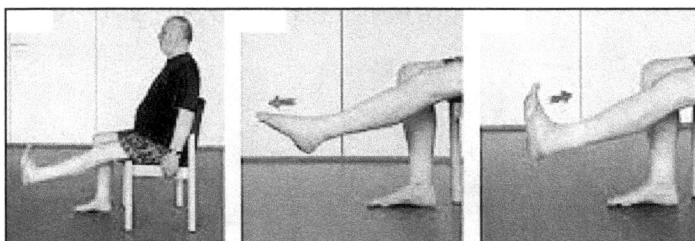

Beginners Legs

Before beginning, please make sure you have all of the items and equipment that is needed. This will require a chair for sitting. Are you ready? Let's get started...

The Beginners Legs is for the Senior/Elderly who is able to do leg exercises. Below, I have provided a couple of exercises just for you. They are very simple and as you continue to do them, you may even move up to the

Immediate Level very soon. The goal is to move up to the highest level. I encourage you to do your best and please do it with a positive attitude as you increase your faith and determination. You may have an assistant or you may do these by yourself. Take your time, you do not have to rush, rushing will only injure you. But, when you take your time and do them right, it will be rewarding for you. Just do not quit. You can do it... Let's go!

Items Needed:

1. Sweat towel
2. Walking shoes
3. Socks
4. Shorts or warm ups
5. T-Shirt or comfortable shirt
6. A chair, matt, or large towel
7. You may listen to music as you do this

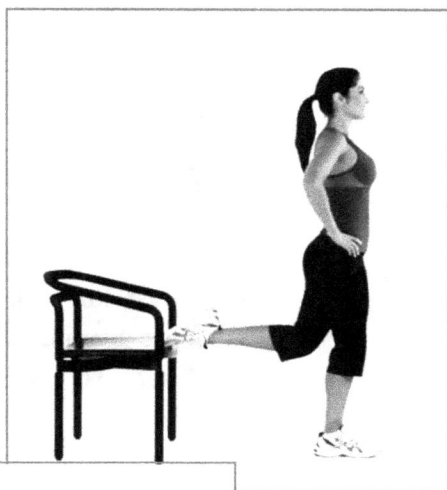

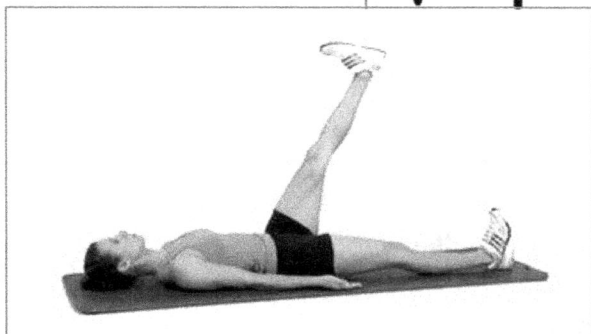

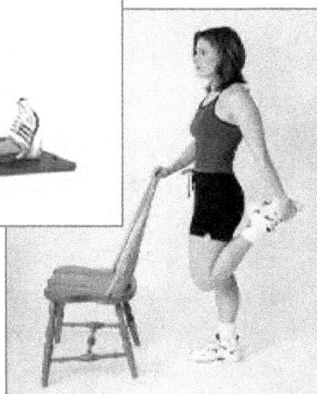

| REMEMBER | Stand strong or sit tall as you use your legs and do not lock your knees. Control your breathing as you inhale through your nose, and exhale through your mouth. Follow the instructions for the Leg Exercises on the next page. |

START EXERCISES

✓ BEGINNERS LEGS

1. **EXERCISE 1:** You will stand behind a chair and bend your right and left leg upward one at a time for either a 3-5 count or a 5-10 count, whichever one is best for you. You will then rest for 30-seconds to 1 minute. You will repeat this process for 3-5 sets. You will repeat this process for 3-5 days. You may extend the days if desire. If you desire to extend your days, you will need to increase the amount of times on each exercise each week you continue.

2. **EXERCISE 2:** You will stand behind a chair as you hold on to the back of the chair for support, and extend your left and right leg to the left and to the right. You will then squat down as you bend your knees and thrust back upward. You are encouraged to bend your knees as low as you can. You will do this for a 5-10 count. You will rest for 1 minute. You will do this for 3-5 sets. You will repeat this process for both exercises for 3-5 days. You may extend the days if desire. If you desire to extend your days, you will need to increase the amount of times on each exercise each week you continue.

Immediate Legs

The Immediate Legs is for the Senior/Elderly who is able to walk but your strength will not allow you to for a medium to long distance. I have provided a couple of exercises just for you below. They are very simple and as you continue to do them, you may even move up to the Senior Pro Level very soon. The goal is to move up to the highest level. I encourage you to do your best and please do it with a positive attitude as you increase your faith and determination. You may have an assistant or you may do these by yourself. Take your time, you do not have to rush, rushing will only injure you. But, when you take your time and do them right, it will be rewarding for you. Just do not quit. You can do it... Let's go!

Items Needed:
1. Sweat towel
2. Walking shoes
3. Socks
4. Shorts or warm ups
5. T-Shirt or comfortable shirt
6. Large matt or large towel
7. You may listen to music as you do this

START EXERCISES

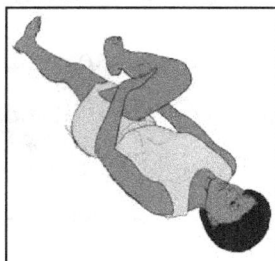

✓ IMMEDIATE LEGS

1. **EXERCISE 1:** You will stand and straddle your legs as wide as you can. You will then lunge to the right then to the left as far as you can as your hands are on your waist. You will repeat this process 5-8 times and will rest for 1-2 minutes. You will repeat the process again for a total of 3-5 sets. You will repeat this process for 3-5 days. You may extend the days if desire. If you desire to extend your days, you will need to increase the amount of times on each exercise each week you continue.

2. **EXERCISE2:** You will stand straight up with your hands to your side. You will then lift your right and alternate with your left leg upward (like a knee high) as high as you can for 5-10 count. You will do this for a 3-5 sets.

Senior Pro Legs

The Senior Pro Legs is for the Senior/Elderly who is able to power walk for a long distance. Power walking is walking at a fast rate of speed. It is almost like running but you are still in a fast walking mode. I have provided a couple of exercises just for you below. They are very simple and as you continue to do them, you may even want to increase your walking distance and minutes very soon. The goal is to go higher and higher. I encourage you to do your best and please do it with a positive attitude as you increase your faith and determination. You may have an assistant or you may do these by yourself. Take your time, you do not have to rush, rushing will only injure you. But, when you take your time and do them right, it will be rewarding for you. Just do not quit. You can do it... Let's go!

Items Needed:
1. Sweat towel
2. Walking shoes
3. Socks
4. Shorts or warm ups
5. T-Shirt or comfortable shirt
6. Large Matt or large towel
7. You may listen to music as you do this

START EXERCISES

✓ SENIOR PRO LEGS

1. **EXERCISE:** You will sit in a chair with your hands on your waist as you extend your legs straight out and back down to the floor and then immediately stand up, and then sit right back down. You will repeat this process for 10-15 times. You will also repeat the process for 3-5 sets. You may increase the amount of times and the sets as you get stronger or as needed.

2. **EXERCISE 2:** You will stand in front of a chair, place both hands on the seat of the chair, extend your right and then your left leg backward as far as you can for 5-10 times. You will repeat this for 3-5 sets. You will repeat both exercises for 3-5 days. You may extend the days if desire. If you desire to extend your days, you will need to increase the amount of times and sets on each exercise each week you continue.

Now that you have completed the Legs Exercises and got your starting experience, you should challenge yourself to go a little further by starting and finishing The 5-Week Exercise & Eating Plan located in Chapter 6. I encourage you to start and finish it successfully.

CHAPTER 5

The Eating Plan

Experience the New Re*shaped* YOU

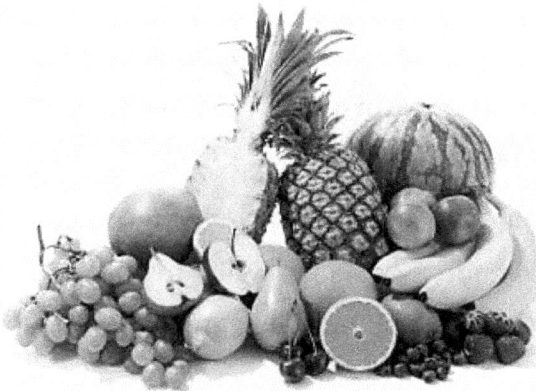

Practically everyone is concerned about getting older. Weight, having good health, and a consistent exercise plan that fits you is what comes to mind. No one wants to gain weight and have to deal with being overweight. No one wants to deal with their bones and muscles giving out on them. No one wants to deal with not having enough strength to last all day and each day. As you get older, there is generally a decline in muscle strength and flexibility. By making wise food choices and monitoring portion sizes, drinking plenty of water, increasing physical activity (strength, flexibility, aerobic training along with your daily activities), and closely watching your posture, you can slow the aging process.

As one intake fatty meals, the body increases fatty tissues. Fatty acids absorb and transport to the liver, where essential nutrients are removed. The rest are packaged together with proteins to form chylomicrons, so that it can travel throughout the bloodstream to all the organs and cells that need it. This is why it is important not to eat fatty foods. If you eat more fat than the body needs, it either gets stored in the arteries of your heart—which is not a good thing, or it can also can get stored in your liver—which can give you a fatty liver, and can spread to your hips, thighs, buttocks, or abdomen; which is also not a good thing.

Are you ready to be REshaped? Have you gone through each chapter and the process in this book to experience the NEW REshaped YOU? I can tell you it feels great to experience the NEW REshaped YOU. The only example I can give is when you first step out of a hot bubble bath, the cleansing you feel after you have washed off the old dirt and grim from the stress of the day, and put on the NEW REshaped YOU, a clean NEW look, the feeling you feel is far better than what the example can give.

You no longer feel heavy and bound. You no longer feel like your limbs can't move or go any further. Your bones feel active. You don't feel weak and as if you're falling. You don't feel uncoordinated or imbalanced. Your mind and spirit is free from doubt and you feel motivated within to live a healthy life through exercise and healthy eating. You feel light and a NEW YOU. You no longer feel sad, lonely, discouraged, and hurt about situations that may have caused you not to want to exercise, eat healthy, and feel happy and full of life. You have made a choice to live again and leave your negative past behind. This is what I mean by experiencing the NEW REshaped YOU. I encourage you to experience it today!

Below, I have given you a detailed eating plan suggestion as you experience the NEW REshaped YOU.

✓ Weight Loss Eating Plan Question:

You may ask the question, "how much should I weigh?" I will answer, with a proper eating plan, you should weigh the proper weight for your height.

With a weight loss diet/eating plan, you can lower your blood pressure, blood sugar (diabetes), and risk of heart decease.

✓ Here is a Weight Loss Eating Plan Suggestion Below:

Stay away from white breads as much as possible (wheat breads recommended only if eating bread).

Weight loss can come through a low-carbohydrate diet/eating plan. This can prevent many health conditions and issues. If followed, it can reduce the risk of health issues.

✓ Weight Loss Eating Plan

You may ask the question, "how can I get and feel healthy at my age?" I will answer by making sure you abide by a proper diet and daily exercise. You want to stay as active as you can. Watch your food intake. You do not have to eat every meal until you are stuffed full and can hardly move.

This will only blow you up and pretty soon if repeated daily will put immediate pounds on you. Eat a balance meal as you do not seek to get full, but eat just enough to get you to your next meal while drinking plenty of water. I encourage you to follow the 5-Week Exercise & Eating Plan in chapter 6. This will give you an idea of what you should eat and how much you should be eating on a daily basis.

Below is how your diet/eating plan should be set up as you put the right foods together and remove the wrong foods that hinder.

Here's How it Works:
Low-Carbohydrate Diet below-
- Protein
- Vegetables
- Healthy fat

Whole Grains-
- Barley
- Oaks
- Rice

Forbidden Foods You Should <u>Not</u> Eat-
- White sugar
- White rice
- White bread
- White potatoes

- Pasta made with flour
- Starchy vegetables
- Dairy products

Your goal should be to rev up your body's ability to burn fat. As you lose the weight, you can add some carbohydrates back into your diet/eating plan such as:

- Berries
- Yogurt
- Nuts
- Fruits

Your goal should be to stick to the diet/eating plan until you are at your desired weight. This should encourage you to stick to your diet/eating plan and keep your weight at the desired weight you are wanting and needing.

With a daily healthy eating plan, you can increase your chances of <u>not</u> getting diabetes, high cholesterol, clogged arteries, high blood pressure, other diseases, and weak bones and muscles due to lack of nourishment.

For more detailed information on eating healthy, you may purchase my book "REshape YOU: *A Guide to Teach YOU How to Create the NEW YOU from the Inside Out.*"

CHAPTER 6
The 5-Week Exercises & Eating Plan

This point in the book is where my **5-Week Exercises and Eating** Plan begins. It provides you a step-by-step exercise and eating plan instruction on how you should successfully complete each day and week until the 5-week plans are completed.

You should complete each exercise 3-5 days per week. You can repeat exercises more than 3 days if your ability and strength allows. You may also start with less days until you become stronger. However, a proper rest is required within each week.

You should be aware before beginning that each exercise may be too rigorous if you are just beginning. Please begin the exercise plan carefully while taking your time. If you believe the exercise plan is too rigorous for you, please consult your physician before beginning.

You are encouraged to work with a partner or with a group. However, exercising alone works just the same. Please read the instructions on the next page before beginning.

Raedy? Let's get started...

WEEK 1
DATE: _____

It is recommended that
you stretch before
beginning exercises
each day.

STRETCHING LOG SHEET

STRETCHING	DAY 1	DAY 2	DAY 3
Complete 3-sets of 10-15 second count for each stretch	Place a ✓ check in the appropriate box to show you have completed the stretch successfully for each day.		
TOE TOUCHES			
LUNGES TO RIGHT AND LEFT			
NECK ROLL: *ROLL NECK ROUND AND ROUND*			
RIGHT AND LEFT ARM BEND EXTENTION: *BEND ARM BEHIND HEAD AND PULL WITH OPPOSITE HAND THE OPPOSITE DIRECTION*			
RIGHT AND LEFT ARM STRAIGHT EXTENTION: *EXTEND ARM STRAIGHT ACROSS NECK AND HOLD WITH OPPOSITE HAND*			

It is recommended that you count out loud to keep count.

EXERCISE
LOG SHEET

EXERCISE	DAY 1	DAY 2	DAY 3
Complete 3-sets of 10 repetitions for each exercise	Place a ✓ check in the appropriate box to show you have completed the exercise successfully for each day.		
KICK-OUTS			
KICK TAPS			
SQUATS			
TOE TOUCHES: *BEND DOWN AND TOUCH TOES*			
STANDING WALL PUSH-UPS			
WALK IN PLACE OR OUTSIDE FOR 1, 2, 3, OR 5 MINUTES			
SEATED LEG LIFTS			
SEATED ARM LIFTS: *IN FRONT AND ON SIDES*			

I have designed sitting exercises for those who are unable to stand or stand long. See Sitting <u>Only</u> Exercise Log Sheet below.

SITTING <u>ONLY</u> EXERCISE LOG SHEET

EXERCISE	DAY 1	DAY 2	DAY 3
Complete 3-sets of 10 repetitions for each exercise	Place a ✓check in the appropriate box to show you have completed the exercise successfully for each day.		
SEATED LEG LIFTS			
KICK TAPS			
BEND OVERS: *BEND AND TOUCH TOES*			
KNEE TOUCHES: *ALTERNATE TOUCHING KNEES AND CHEST*			
SITTING AIR PUSHES: *PUSH ARMS STRAIGHT OUTWARD AND BACK*			
SEATED ARM LIFTS: *IN FRONT AND ON SIDES*			

I have designed bed exercises for those who are unable to stand or get out of bed. See Bed Exercise Log Sheet below.

BED EXERCISE
LOG SHEET

EXERCISE	DAY 1	DAY 2	DAY 3
Complete 3-sets of 3 or 5 repetitions for each exercise	Place a ✓check in the appropriate box to show you have completed the exercise successfully for each day.		
ARM LIFTS: *ALTERNATE LIFTING ARMS TO THE SKY*			
ARM CURLS: *ALTERNATE CURLING EACH ARM TOWARD CHECT AND DOWN*			
BODY LIFTS: *LIFT BODY UP TO A SITTING POSITION AND BACK DOWN*			
TOE WIGGLES: *WIGGLE TOES AS FAST AS YOU CAN FOR 3-5 SECONDS*			
LEG LIFTS: *ALTERNATE LIFTING LEGS STRAIGHT UP AND DOWN*			

WEEK 1 *REVIEW*

Now that you have completed week 1. I have provided a few questions for improvement. Also, you may write additional exercises and/or activities you have completed. Write them down on the chart located on the next page.

QUESTIONS:

HOW DO YOU FEEL AFTER COMPLETING WEEK 1? WHY?

WERE YOU ABLE TO COMPLETE EACH EXERCISE?

DID YOU GET TIRED AFTER THE FIRST EXERCISE?

WERE YOU ABLE TO DO EACH REPETITION?

DID YOU NEED REST TIME IN BETWEEN EACH EXERCISE?

ARE YOU EMPOWERED TO COMPLETE THE FULL 5-WEEK EXERCISE PLAN? IF SO, WHY OR WHY NOT?

EXERCISES/ACTIVITES	DESCRIPTION
EX. *Biking*	*Rode bikes in the park for 1 hour. Got more strength.*

ADDITIONAL PERSONAL NOTES

_____

_____

_____

_____

_____

_____

_____

_____

_____

_____

_____

_____

_____

_____

TAKE THE WEEK 1 EXERCISE CHALLENGE

Challenge #1
Challenge yourself to eat healthy.

Challenge #2
Be persistent and consistent in each exercise. Complete each repetition for full maximum results. Do not become weary now that you have first begun. Your body may be sore and may feel tired, but do not quit. Your improvement may not show on the outside yet, but if you keep going, you will begin to see results in your health and in your body real soon.

Challenge #3
Exercise on every assigned day and have faith in yourself.

Challenge #4
Experience the **RE*shaped* NEW YOU** from the inside out—feeling great, looking great from the inside out!

POWER NOTES:

Add your comment if you have already experienced a change.

POWER NOTE 1

1. As you get stronger, you may add ankle and arm weights with your exercise for greater maximum results.

POWER NOTE 2

2. Go into each exercise strong, expecting positive results.

POWER NOTE 3

3. You may increase your repetitions on each exercise as the weeks increase for maximum results.

POWER NOTE 4

4. BELIEVE IN YOURSELF.

POWER NOTE 5

5. If you choose to add additional exercises and activities, you should be just as motivated as you are with the REshape YOU exercises.

POWER NOTE 6

6. Motivate your faith and be positive and not negative.

WEEK 2
DATE: _____

It is recommended that
you stretch before
beginning exercises
each day.

STRETCHING LOG SHEET

STRETCHING	DAY 1	DAY 2	DAY 3
Complete 3-sets of 10-15 second count for each stretch	Place a ✓ check in the appropriate box to show you have completed the stretch successfully for each day.		
TOE TOUCHES			
LUNGES TO RIGHT AND LEFT			
NECK ROLL: *ROLL NECK ROUND AND ROUND*			
RIGHT AND LEFT ARM BEND EXTENTION: *BEND ARM BEHIND HEAD AND PULL WITH OPPOSITE HAND THE OPPOSITE DIRECTION*			
RIGHT AND LEFT ARM STRAIGHT EXTENTION: *EXTEND ARM STRAIGHT ACROSS NECK AND HOLD WITH OPPOSITE HAND*			

It is recommended that you count out loud to keep count.

EXERCISE
LOG SHEET

EXERCISE	DAY 1	DAY 2	DAY 3
Complete 3-sets of 10 repetitions for each exercise	Place a ✓ check in the appropriate box to show you have completed the exercise successfully for each day.		
KICK-OUTS			
KICK TAPS			
SQUATS			
TOE TOUCHES: *BEND DOWN AND TOUCH TOES*			
STANDING WALL PUSH-UPS			
WALK IN PLACE OR OUTSIDE FOR 1, 2, 3, OR 5 MINUTES			
SEATED LEG LIFTS			
SEATED ARM LIFTS: *IN FRONT AND ON SIDES*			

I have designed sitting exercises for those who are unable to stand or stand long. See Sitting <u>Only</u> Exercise Log Sheet below.

SITTING <u>ONLY</u> EXERCISE LOG SHEET

EXERCISE	DAY 1	DAY 2	DAY 3
Complete 3-sets of 10 repetitions for each exercise	Place a ✓check in the appropriate box to show you have completed the exercise successfully for each day.		
SEATED LEG LIFTS			
KICK TAPS			
BEND OVERS: *BEND AND TOUCH TOES*			
KNEE TOUCHES: *ALTERNATE TOUCHING KNEES AND CHEST*			
SITTING AIR PUSHES: *PUSH ARMS STRAIGHT OUTWARD AND BACK*			
SEATED ARM LIFTS: *IN FRONT AND ON SIDES*			

I have designed bed exercises for those who are unable to stand or get out of bed. See Bed Exercise Log Sheet below.

BED EXERCISE

LOG SHEET

EXERCISE	DAY 1	DAY 2	DAY 3
Complete 3-sets of 3 or 5 repetitions for each exercise	Place a ✓check in the appropriate box to show you have completed the exercise successfully for each day.		
ARM LIFTS: *ALTERNATE LIFTING ARMS TO THE SKY*			
ARM CURLS: *ALTERNATE CURLING EACH ARM TOWARD CHECT AND DOWN*			
BODY LIFTS: *LIFT BODY UP TO A SITTING POSITION AND BACK DOWN*			
TOE WIGGLES: *WIGGLE TOES AS FAST AS YOU CAN FOR 3-5 SECONDS*			
LEG LIFTS: *ALTERNATE LIFTING LEGS STRAIGHT UP AND DOWN*			

WEEK 2 *REVIEW*

Now that you have completed week 2. I have provided a few questions for improvement. Also, you may write additional exercises and/or activities you have completed. Write them down on the chart below.

QUESTIONS:

HOW DO YOU FEEL AFTER COMPLETING WEEK 2? WHY?

WERE YOU ABLE TO COMPLETE EACH EXERCISE?

DID YOU GET TIRED AFTER THE FIRST EXERCISE?

DO YOU FEEL A LITTLE STRONGER? WHY OR WHY NOT?

DID YOU NEED REST TIME IN BETWEEN EACH EXERCISE?

ARE YOU EMPOWERED TO COMPLETE THE FULL 5-WEEK EXERCISE PLAN? IF SO, WHY OR WHY NOT?

EXERCISES/ACTIVITES	DESCRIPTION
EX. *Biking*	*Rode bikes in the park for 1 hour. Got more strength.*

ADDITIONAL PERSONAL NOTES

_____

_____

_____

_____

_____

_____

_____

_____

_____

_____

_____

_____

_____

_____

_____

TAKE THE WEEK 2 EXERCISE CHALLENGE

Challenge #1
Challenge yourself to eat healthy.

Challenge #2
Be persistent and consistent in each exercise. Complete each repetition for full maximum results. Do not become weary in your second week. Your body may be sore and may feel tired, but do not quit. Your improvement may not show on the outside yet, but if you keep going, you will begin to see results in your health and in your body real soon. DO NOT QUIT. STAY MOTIVATED!

Challenge #3
Exercise on every assigned day and have faith in yourself.

Challenge #4
Experience the **RE*shaped* NEW YOU** from the inside out—feeling great, looking great from the inside out!

POWER NOTES:

Add your comment if you have already experienced a change.

POWER NOTE 1

1. As you get stronger, you may add ankle and arm weights with your exercise for greater maximum results.

POWER NOTE 2

2. Go into each exercise strong, expecting positive results.

POWER NOTE 3

3. You may increase your repetitions on each exercise as the weeks increase for maximum results.

POWER NOTE 4

4. BELIEVE IN YOURSELF.

POWER NOTE 5

5. If you choose to add additional exercises and activities, you should be just as motivated as you are with the REshape YOU exercises.

POWER NOTE 6

6. Motivate your faith and be positive and not negative.

WEEK 3
DATE: _____

It is recommended that
you stretch before
beginning exercises
each day.

STRETCHING LOG SHEET

STRETCHING	DAY 1	DAY 2	DAY 3
Complete 3-sets of 10-15 second count for each stretch	Place a ✓ check in the appropriate box to show you have completed the stretch successfully for each day.		
TOE TOUCHES			
LUNGES TO RIGHT AND LEFT			
NECK ROLL: *ROLL NECK ROUND AND ROUND*			
RIGHT AND LEFT ARM BEND EXTENTION: *BEND ARM BEHIND HEAD AND PULL WITH OPPOSITE HAND THE OPPOSITE DIRECTION*			
RIGHT AND LEFT ARM STRAIGHT EXTENTION: *EXTEND ARM STRAIGHT ACROSS NECK AND HOLD WITH OPPOSITE HAND*			

It is recommended that you count out loud to keep count.

EXERCISE
LOG SHEET

EXERCISE	DAY 1	DAY 2	DAY 3
Complete 3-sets of 10 repetitions for each exercise	Place a ✓ check in the appropriate box to show you have completed the exercise successfully for each day.		
KICK-OUTS			
KICK TAPS			
SQUATS			
TOE TOUCHES: *BEND DOWN AND TOUCH TOES*			
STANDING WALL PUSH-UPS			
WALK IN PLACE OR OUTSIDE FOR 1, 2, 3, OR 5 MINUTES			
SEATED LEG LIFTS			
SEATED ARM LIFTS: *IN FRONT AND ON SIDES*			

I have designed sitting exercises for those who are unable to stand or stand long. See Sitting <u>Only</u> Exercise Log Sheet below.

SITTING <u>ONLY</u> EXERCISE LOG SHEET

EXERCISE	DAY 1	DAY 2	DAY 3
Complete 3-sets of 10 repetitions for each exercise	Place a ✓check in the appropriate box to show you have completed the exercise successfully for each day.		
SEATED LEG LIFTS			
KICK TAPS			
BEND OVERS: *BEND AND TOUCH TOES*			
KNEE TOUCHES: *ALTERNATE TOUCHING KNEES AND CHEST*			
SITTING AIR PUSHES: *PUSH ARMS STRAIGHT OUTWARD AND BACK*			
SEATED ARM LIFTS: *IN FRONT AND ON SIDES*			

I have designed bed exercises for those who are unable to stand or get out of bed. See Bed Exercise Log Sheet below.

BED EXERCISE
LOG SHEET

EXERCISE	DAY 1	DAY 2	DAY 3
Complete 3-sets of 3 or 5 repetitions for each exercise	Place a ✓check in the appropriate box to show you have completed the exercise successfully for each day.		
ARM LIFTS: *ALTERNATE LIFTING ARMS TO THE SKY*			
ARM CURLS: *ALTERNATE CURLING EACH ARM TOWARD CHECT AND DOWN*			
BODY LIFTS: *LIFT BODY UP TO A SITTING POSITION AND BACK DOWN*			
TOE WIGGLES: *WIGGLE TOES AS FAST AS YOU CAN FOR 3-5 SECONDS*			
LEG LIFTS: *ALTERNATE LIFTING LEGS STRAIGHT UP AND DOWN*			

WEEK 3 *REVIEW*

Now that you have completed week 3. I have provided a few questions for improvement. Also, you may write additional exercises and/or activities you have completed. Write them down on the chart below.

QUESTIONS:

HOW DO YOU FEEL AFTER COMPLETING WEEK 3? WHY?

WERE YOU ABLE TO COMPLETE EACH EXERCISE?

DID YOU GET TIRED AFTER THE FIRST EXERCISE?

DO YOU FEEL STRONGER? WHY OR WHY NOT?

DID YOU NEED REST TIME IN BETWEEN EACH EXERCISE?

ARE YOU EMPOWERED TO COMPLETE THE FULL 5-WEEK EXERCISE PLAN? IF SO, WHY OR WHY NOT?

EXERCISES/ACTIVITES	DESCRIPTION
EX. *Biking*	*Rode bikes in the park for 1 hour. Got more strength.*

ADDITIONAL PERSONAL NOTES

TAKE THE WEEK 3 EXERCISE CHALLENGE

Challenge #1
Challenge yourself to eat healthy as you follow the eating plan I have provided, and stay consistent with each day of exercising.

Challenge #2
Be persistent and consistent in each exercise. Complete each repetition for full maximum results. Do not become weary. DO NOT QUIT. STAY MOTIVATED!

Challenge #3
Exercise on every assigned day and have faith in yourself.

Challenge #4
Experience the **RE*shaped* NEW YOU** from the inside out—feeling great, looking great from the inside out!

POWER NOTES:

Add your comment if you have already experienced a change.

POWER NOTE 1

1. As you get stronger, you may add ankle and arm weights with your exercise for greater maximum results.

POWER NOTE 2

2. Go into each exercise strong, expecting positive results.

POWER NOTE 3

3. You may increase your repetitions on each exercise as the weeks increase for maximum results.

POWER NOTE 4

4. BELIEVE IN YOURSELF.

POWER NOTE 5

5. If you choose to add additional exercises and activities, you should be just as motivated as you are with the REshape YOU exercises.

POWER NOTE 6

6. Motivate your faith and be positive and not negative.

WEEK 4
DATE: _____

It is recommended that
you stretch before
beginning exercises
each day.

STRETCHING LOG SHEET

STRETCHING	DAY 1	DAY 2	DAY 3
Complete 3-sets of 10-15 second count for each stretch	Place a ✓ check in the appropriate box to show you have completed the stretch successfully for each day.		
TOE TOUCHES			
LUNGES TO RIGHT AND LEFT			
NECK ROLL: *ROLL NECK ROUND AND ROUND*			
RIGHT AND LEFT ARM BEND EXTENTION: *BEND ARM BEHIND HEAD AND PULL WITH OPPOSITE HAND THE OPPOSITE DIRECTION*			
RIGHT AND LEFT ARM STRAIGHT EXTENTION: *EXTEND ARM STRAIGHT ACROSS NECK AND HOLD WITH OPPOSITE HAND*			

It is recommended that you count out loud to keep count.

EXERCISE
LOG SHEET

EXERCISE	DAY 1	DAY 2	DAY 3
Complete 3-sets of 10 repetitions for each exercise	Place a ✓ check in the appropriate box to show you have completed the exercise successfully for each day.		
KICK-OUTS			
KICK TAPS			
SQUATS			
TOE TOUCHES: *BEND DOWN AND TOUCH TOES*			
STANDING WALL PUSH-UPS			
WALK IN PLACE OR OUTSIDE FOR 1, 2, 3, OR 5 MINUTES			
SEATED LEG LIFTS			
SEATED ARM LIFTS: *IN FRONT AND ON SIDES*			

I have designed sitting exercises for those who are unable to stand or stand long. See Sitting <u>Only</u> Exercise Log Sheet below.

SITTING <u>ONLY</u> EXERCISE LOG SHEET

EXERCISE	DAY 1	DAY 2	DAY 3
Complete 3-sets of 10 repetitions for each exercise	Place a ✓ check in the appropriate box to show you have completed the exercise successfully for each day.		
SEATED LEG LIFTS			
KICK TAPS			
BEND OVERS: *BEND AND TOUCH TOES*			
KNEE TOUCHES: *ALTERNATE TOUCHING KNEES AND CHEST*			
SITTING AIR PUSHES: *PUSH ARMS STRAIGHT OUTWARD AND BACK*			
SEATED ARM LIFTS: *IN FRONT AND ON SIDES*			

I have designed bed exercises for those who are unable to stand or get out of bed. See Bed Exercise Log Sheet below.

BED EXERCISE
LOG SHEET

EXERCISE	DAY 1	DAY 2	DAY 3
Complete 3-sets of 3 or 5 repetitions for each exercise	Place a ✓check in the appropriate box to show you have completed the exercise successfully for each day.		
ARM LIFTS: *ALTERNATE LIFTING ARMS TO THE SKY*			
ARM CURLS: *ALTERNATE CURLING EACH ARM TOWARD CHECT AND DOWN*			
BODY LIFTS: *LIFT BODY UP TO A SITTING POSITION AND BACK DOWN*			
TOE WIGGLES: *WIGGLE TOES AS FAST AS YOU CAN FOR 3-5 SECONDS*			
LEG LIFTS: *ALTERNATE LIFTING LEGS STRAIGHT UP AND DOWN*			

WEEK 4 *REVIEW*

Now that you have completed week 4. I have provided a few questions for improvement. Also, you may write additional exercises and/or activities you have completed. Write them down on the chart below.

QUESTIONS:

HOW DO YOU FEEL AFTER COMPLETING WEEK 4? WHY?

WERE YOU ABLE TO COMPLETE EACH EXERCISE?

DID YOU GET TIRED AFTER THE FIRST EXERCISE?

WERE YOU ABLE TO DO EACH REPETITION SUCCESSFULLY?

DID YOU NEED REST TIME IN BETWEEN EACH EXERCISE?

ARE YOU EMPOWERED TO COMPLETE THE FULL 5-WEEK EXERCISE PLAN? IF SO, WHY OR WHY NOT?

EXERCISES/ACTIVITES	DESCRIPTION
EX. *Biking*	*Rode bikes in the park for 1 hour. Got more strength.*

ADDITIONAL PERSONAL NOTES

TAKE THE WEEK 4 EXERCISE CHALLENGE

Challenge #1
Challenge yourself to eat healthy as you follow the eating plan I have provided, and stay consistent with each day of exercising.

Challenge #2
Be persistent and consistent in each exercise. Complete each repetition for full maximum results. Do not become weary. DO NOT QUIT. STAY MOTIVATED!

Challenge #3
Exercise on every assigned day and have faith in yourself.

Challenge #4
Experience the **RE*shaped* NEW YOU** from the inside out— feeling great, looking great from the inside out!

POWER NOTES:

Add your comment if you have already experienced a change.

POWER NOTE 1

1. As you get stronger, you may add ankle and arm weights with your exercise for greater maximum results.

POWER NOTE 2

2. Go into each exercise strong, expecting positive results.

POWER NOTE 3

3. You may increase your repetitions on each exercise as the weeks increase for maximum results.

POWER NOTE 4

4. BELIEVE IN YOURSELF.

POWER NOTE 5

5. If you choose to add additional exercises and activities, you should be just as motivated as you are with the REshape YOU exercises.

POWER NOTE 6

6. Motivate your faith and be positive and not negative.

WEEK 5
DATE: _____

It is recommended that
you stretch before
beginning exercises
each day.

STRETCHING LOG SHEET

STRETCHING	DAY 1	DAY 2	DAY 3
Complete 3-sets of 10-15 second count for each stretch	Place a ✓ check in the appropriate box to show you have completed the stretch successfully for each day.		
TOE TOUCHES			
LUNGES TO RIGHT AND LEFT			
NECK ROLL: *ROLL NECK ROUND AND ROUND*			
RIGHT AND LEFT ARM BEND EXTENTION: *BEND ARM BEHIND HEAD AND PULL WITH OPPOSITE HAND THE OPPOSITE DIRECTION*			
RIGHT AND LEFT ARM STRAIGHT EXTENTION: *EXTEND ARM STRAIGHT ACROSS NECK AND HOLD WITH OPPOSITE HAND*			

It is recommended that you count out loud to keep count.

EXERCISE
LOG SHEET

EXERCISE	DAY 1	DAY 2	DAY 3
Complete 3-sets of 10 repetitions for each exercise	Place a ✓ check in the appropriate box to show you have completed the exercise successfully for each day.		
KICK-OUTS			
KICK TAPS			
SQUATS			
TOE TOUCHES: *BEND DOWN AND TOUCH TOES*			
STANDING WALL PUSH-UPS			
WALK IN PLACE OR OUTSIDE FOR 1, 2, 3, OR 5 MINUTES			
SEATED LEG LIFTS			
SEATED ARM LIFTS: *IN FRONT AND ON SIDES*			

I have designed sitting exercises for those who are unable to stand or stand long. See Sitting <u>Only</u> Exercise Log Sheet below.

SITTING <u>ONLY</u> EXERCISE LOG SHEET

EXERCISE	DAY 1	DAY 2	DAY 3
Complete 3-sets of 10 repetitions for each exercise	Place a ✓check in the appropriate box to show you have completed the exercise successfully for each day.		
SEATED LEG LIFTS			
KICK TAPS			
BEND OVERS: *BEND AND TOUCH TOES*			
KNEE TOUCHES: *ALTERNATE TOUCHING KNEES AND CHEST*			
SITTING AIR PUSHES: *PUSH ARMS STRAIGHT OUTWARD AND BACK*			
SEATED ARM LIFTS: *IN FRONT AND ON SIDES*			

I have designed bed exercises for those who are unable to stand or get out of bed. See Bed Exercise Log Sheet below.

BED EXERCISE
LOG SHEET

EXERCISE	DAY 1	DAY 2	DAY 3
Complete 3-sets of 3 or 5 repetitions for each exercise	Place a ✓check in the appropriate box to show you have completed the exercise successfully for each day.		
ARM LIFTS: *ALTERNATE LIFTING ARMS TO THE SKY*			
ARM CURLS: *ALTERNATE CURLING EACH ARM TOWARD CHECT AND DOWN*			
BODY LIFTS: *LIFT BODY UP TO A SITTING POSITION AND BACK DOWN*			
TOE WIGGLES: *WIGGLE TOES AS FAST AS YOU CAN FOR 3-5 SECONDS*			
LEG LIFTS: *ALTERNATE LIFTING LEGS STRAIGHT UP AND DOWN*			

WEEK 5 *REVIEW*

Now that you have completed week 5. I have provided a few questions for improvement. Also, you may write additional exercises and/or activities you have completed. Write them down on the chart below.

QUESTIONS:

HOW DO YOU FEEL AFTER COMPLETING WEEK 5? WHY?

WERE YOU ABLE TO COMPLETE EACH EXERCISE? WHY?

WILL YOU REPEAT THE 5-WEEK EXERCISE PLAN AGAIN? WHY? OR WHY NOT?

DO YOU FEEL RESHAPED OR DO YOU FEEL THAT YOU ARE STILL BEING RESHAPED?

WERE YOU ABLE TO DO THE EXERCISES ALONE?

WERE YOU EMPOWERED TO COMPLETE THE FULL 5-WEEK EXERCISE PLAN? IF SO, WHY OR WHY NOT?

EXERCISES/ACTIVITES	DESCRIPTION
EX. *Biking*	*Rode bikes in the park for 1 hour. Got more strength.*

ADDITIONAL PERSONAL NOTES

TAKE THE WEEK 5 EXERCISE CHALLENGE

Challenge #1
Challenge yourself to eat healthy as you follow the eating plan I have provided, and stay consistent with each day of exercising.

Challenge #2
Be persistent and consistent in each exercise. Complete each repetition for full maximum results. Do not become weary. DO NOT QUIT. STAY MOTIVATED!

Challenge #3
Exercise on every assigned day and have faith in yourself.

Challenge #4
Experience the **RE*shaped* NEW YOU** from the inside out—feeling great, looking great from the inside out!

POWER NOTES:

Add your comment if you have already experienced a change.

POWER NOTE 1
1. As you get stronger, you may add ankle and arm weights with your exercise for greater maximum results.

POWER NOTE 2
2. Go into each exercise strong, expecting positive results.

POWER NOTE 3
3. You may increase your repetitions on each exercise as the weeks increase for maximum results.

POWER NOTE 4
4. BELIEVE IN YOURSELF.

POWER NOTE 5
5. If you choose to add additional exercises and activities, you should be just as motivated as you are with the REshape YOU exercises.

POWER NOTE 6
6. Motivate your faith and be positive and not negative.

WEEK 5 *REVIEW*

Now that you have completed week 5. I have provided a few questions for improvement. Also, you may write additional exercises and/or activities you have completed. Write them down on the chart below.

QUESTIONS:

HOW DO YOU FEEL AFTER COMPLETING WEEK 5? WHY?

WERE YOU ABLE TO COMPLETE EACH EXERCISE?

DID YOU GET TIRED AFTER THE FIRST EXERCISE?

WERE YOU ABLE TO DO EACH REPETITION?

DID YOU NEED REST TIME IN BETWEEN EACH EXERCISE?

ARE YOU EMPOWERED TO COMPLETE THE FULL 5-WEEK EXERCISE PLAN? IF SO, WHY OR WHY NOT?

EATING PLAN &
For Daily Use
LOG SHEET

ONE STEP AT A TIME: Remove fat, remove salt, remove sugar, lower sodium, reduce portions (amounts per meal), and add fiber.

MORNING

1. (1) EGG
2. (1) SLICE OF TOAST *(wheat bread, **-OR-** whole wheat bagel (1 ½ ounces).*
3. 1 cup of oatmeal *(quick oats- not instant oats)*
4. For a rushed morning, you may eat cereal that has fiber and no sugar added.
5. (1) juicer/natural fruit drink. *Drink one in the morning, or noon, or night.*
6. (2) 16 oz bottles or cups of water *(must be completed by noon, before lunch).* You may also drink skim milk or a decaffeinated coffee *(optional).*

ADD YOUR PERSONAL NOTES

_____
_____
_____
_____
_____
_____
_____

NOON
1. (1) Sandwich *(wheat bread only with turkey or ham)*.
2. (1) bag of chips preferably "All Natural Chips or Tortilla Chips"*(no salt)*.
3. **-OR-** instead of sandwich and chips, you may do (1 cup) of vegetable soup (unsalted less meat). And saltine crackers *(optional)*
4. (1 cup) of fruit. *Preferably grapes or orange.*
5. (3) 16 oz bottles or cups of water, *or you may drink an unsweet tea (must be completed before dinner).*

ADD YOUR PERSONAL NOTES

_____

_____

_____

NIGHT
1. (1 slice) Baked chicken or turkey
2. (1-2 cups) vegetables *(preferably broccoli, green beans, mixed vegetables)*.
3. (1 cup) of salad *(spinach, pineapple, cucumber, or tuna, or your choice)*.
4. (1 cup) of fruit. Preferably grapes or orange. *(You may also have a choice of (1) banana instead of 1/2 cup of fruit).*
5. (3) 16 oz bottles or cups of water, *or you may drink an unsweet tea (must be completed before bedtime)*

ADD YOUR PERSONAL NOTES

_____

_____

_____

EATING PLAN EACH DAY OF THE WEEK *REVIEW*

I have provided a few questions and a description chart. Write your answers and notes.

QUESTIONS:

HOW DO YOU FEEL AFTER BEGINNING THE EATING PLAN AS YOU HAVE ALREADY BEGUN EXERCISING EACH DAY?

WERE YOU ABLE TO COMPLETE THE EATING PLAN EACH DAY OF THE WEEK? HOW? WAS IT CHALLENGING?

DO YOU FEEL THAT YOU ARE BEING RESHAPED AFTER THE FIRST WEEK TO THE 5TH WEEK?

WERE YOU ABLE TO DRINK PLENTY OF WATER THROUGHOUT THE DAY? WHY OR WHY NOT?

ARE YOU EMPOWERED TO COMPLETE THE FULL 5-WEEK EATING PLAN? IF SO, WHY OR WHY NOT?

ADDITIONAL EATING	DESCRIPTION
EX. *New vegetable*	*I tried celery and made a celery soup.*

ADDITIONAL PERSONAL NOTES

TAKE THE EATING PLAN CHALLENGE

Challenge #1
Challenge yourself to eat healthy.

Challenge #2
Be persistent and consistent in eating vegetables daily.

Challenge #3
Drink plenty of water and juicing.

Challenge #4
Experience the **RE*shaped* NEW YOU** from the inside out.

POWER NOTES:
Add your comment if you have already experienced a change.

POWER NOTE 1
1. As you get stronger, you may add and tweek the eating plan to fit you.

POWER NOTE 2
2. Go into the eating plan strong, expecting positive results.

POWER NOTE 3
3. As the days and weeks increase, and as you are exercising, make sure you follow the eating plan and do not lure off and stop.

POWER NOTE 4
4. BELIEVE IN YOURSELF.

POWER NOTE 5
5. If you choose to add additional food items to your eating plan, please make sure they are not fatty, salty, and sugary food and drink items.

POWER NOTE 6
6. Motivate your faith and be positive and not negative as you experience your **REshape YOU NEW** life.

The REshape YOU Workbook

Set Your Goals

Joint Down Completed Goals

What Diets/Eating plans have you Started?

What Diets/Eating plans have you completed?

Note Pad

CONCLUSION

As we get older our body changes and may not be as fast as it used to be. However, as you exercise on a daily basis along with a daily healthy eating plan, you should be able to feel your younger years stirred up within you, as you will be able to move around better and feel stronger.

While no one's perfect and we all are trying to get where we all need to be, I encourage you to raise the standard within yourself by holding yourself accountable for your health and weight. Run toward the mark to RE*shape* the **NEW YOU**. You will not only feel great, but you will also look great with a completely new determination on the inside and a NEW outlook on life and your future on the outside.

CONTACT ME

Stephanie is a personal trainer, coach, counselor, and motivational speaker. For more information and bookings, and if you would like her to be your Personal Trainer, and/or sign up for her Fitness & Health (group) Boot Camp Program, please email her at:

info@stephaniefranklin.org
reshapeyou.stephaniefranklin.org

In your email, please make sure to add your <u>name</u>, <u>phone</u>, <u>email</u>, and <u>what type of service</u> you would like:

Stephanie Franklin's RE*shape* YOU Fitness & Health:
- Personal Training
- Group Fitness
- Fitness & Health (group) Boot Camp
- Family-Fit-Together
- Teen Fitness
- Kid Fitness
* Elderly Fitness

**Without this information, Stephanie will not be able to return your email.

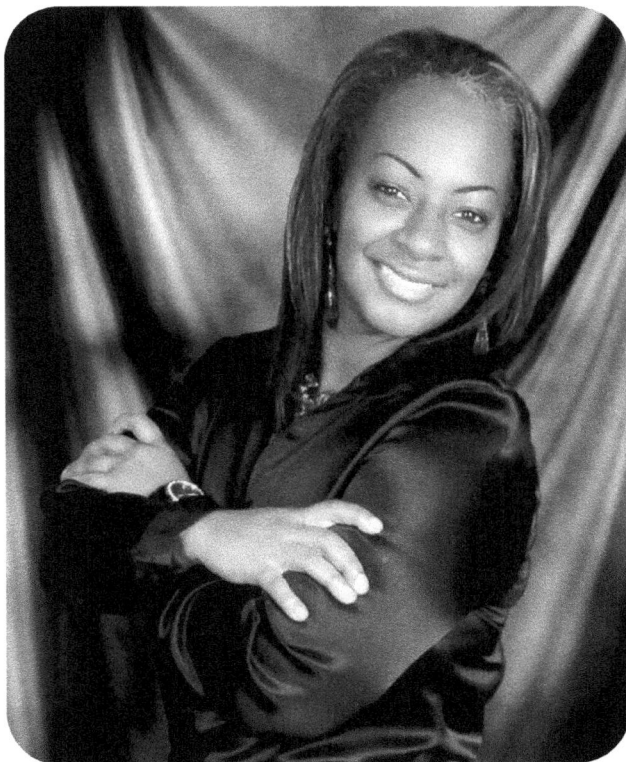

Stephanie Franklin, M.A. (T.H.)

Obtains a Master of Arts degree in Theological Studies and has a vision to reach the world. She has a heart to reach the youth and young adults along with the entire family, bringing them all together as a unified fold. One of her greatest desires is to be used by God in whatever capacity He chooses.